Food For Life

a guide to tube feeding for adults

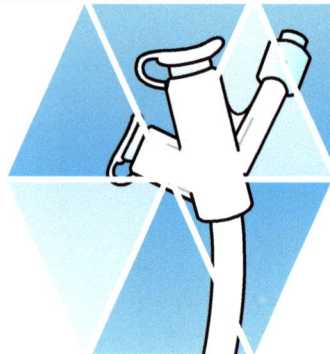

About this book

Food for Life will help you learn how to feed yourself or your loved one through a feeding tube. A feeding tube in the stomach is a G-tube or PEG. A J-tube is a tube in the jejunum (a section of the small intestine)

Caring for yourself with a feeding tube may be a little scary at first. But rest easy. There is little you can do to hurt yourself. With practice, feeding can be simple and comfortable.

In some cases, a person may not be able to understand what the tube is for and may try to pull it out. To prevent this, have him wear bulky mittens, or keep the stoma (the surgical opening) and tube covered with clothes.

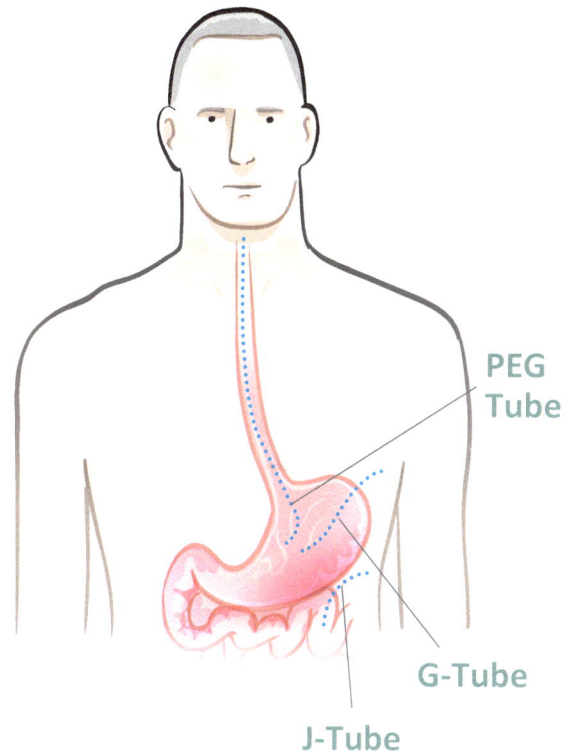

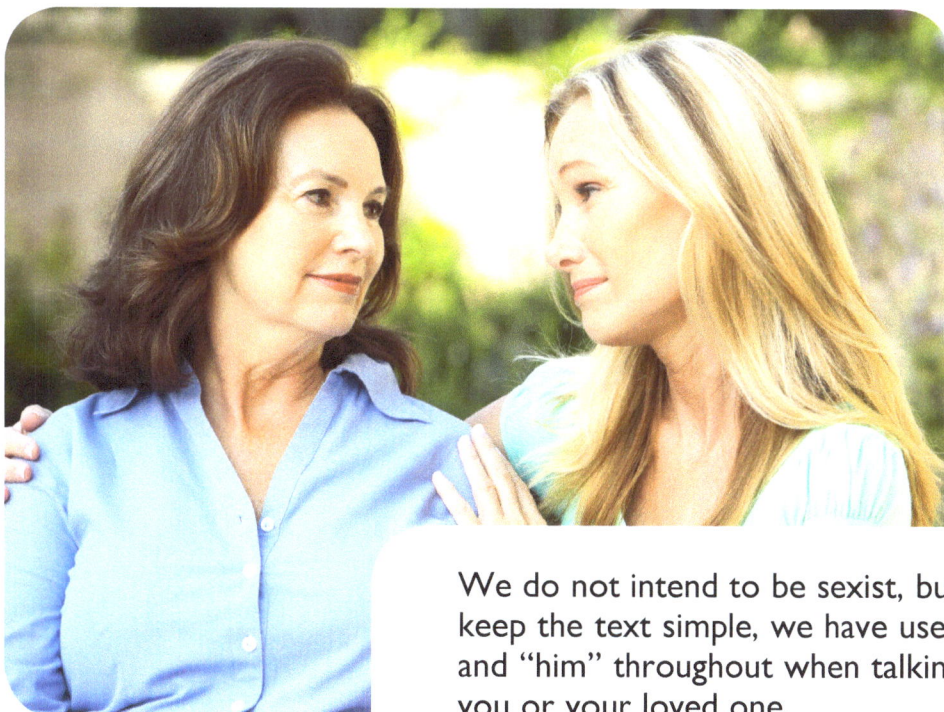

PEG Tube

G-Tube

J-Tube

We do not intend to be sexist, but to keep the text simple, we have used "he" and "him" throughout when talking about you or your loved one.

Feeding tubes

G-tubes, PEG, or J-tubes all have the same **purpose—to give food and medicines** to you if you cannot take them by mouth. They:

- **have ports** (openings)

- **are most often about 12 to 15 inches long** (this is sometimes replaced in a few months with a "button" that lies flat against the abdomen)

- **are placed into the stoma** (the small surgical opening in the belly where the tube enters the stomach or jejunum

- **are kept in place by:**

    – a soft silicone or rubber "bumper" or small balloon (filled with water) inside the stomach

    – a soft rubber or silicone "bumper" (sometimes called a "bolster" or "skin disk" that fits against the skin outside the stoma (This holds the tube in place to keep it from going too far inside the stomach.)

Some tubes are kept in place by using only a balloon or bumper, not both. J-tubes are sometimes sutured in place.

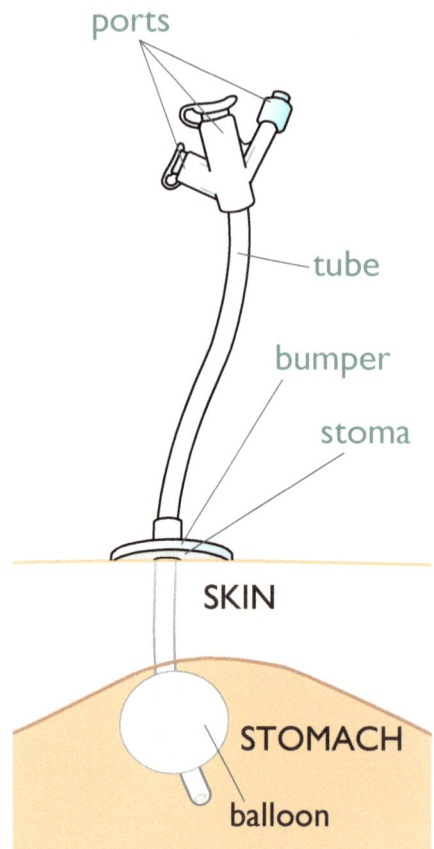

ports

tube

bumper

stoma

SKIN

STOMACH

balloon

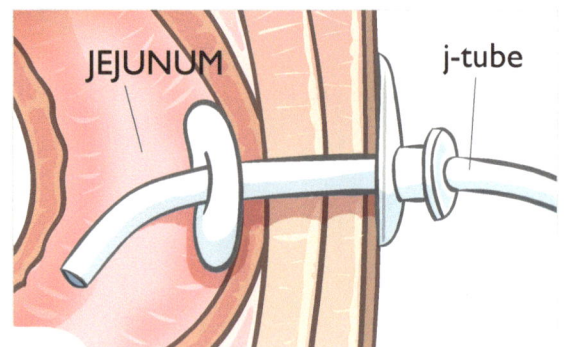

JEJUNUM

j-tube

⊙ CAUTION

If the tube should come out for any reason:

1. place a clean, dry washcloth over the stoma

2. call the doctor or nurse right away

Tube ports are used to give food or medicines or fill the balloon with water. The tube will have 1, 2 or 3 ports.

1-port tubes

Both food and medicines are given through this main port. You will need to flush the tube with warm water before and after giving food and medicines.

2-port tubes

These have a **main feeding port** and a **smaller port.** The main port is used for food and medicines. The smaller port is used one of two ways:

- In tubes with no balloon, it is used to give medicines.

- In tubes with a balloon, it is used to fill the balloon with water.

3-port tubes

- The biggest opening is the feeding port.

- The second port is used for medicines.

- The third port is used to fill the balloon with water.

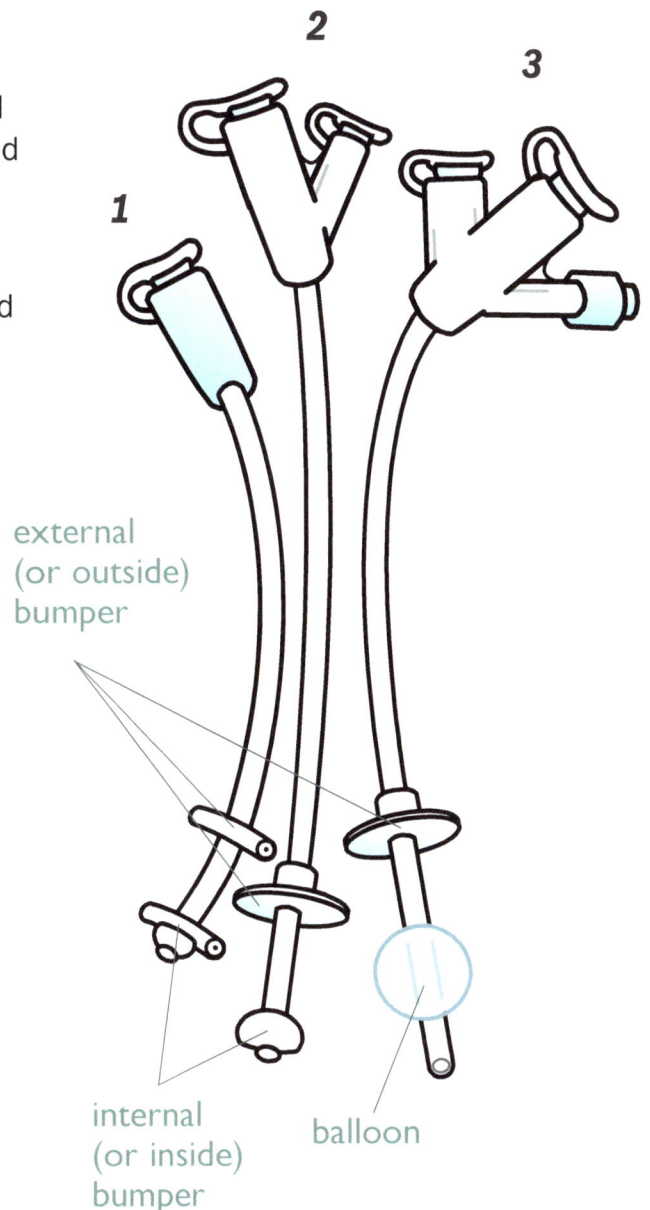

external (or outside) bumper

internal (or inside) bumper

balloon

Most ports have a flip-top cap that must be **closed off when not in use.** (Ports used to fill the balloon with water don't have a cap.)

Ask the doctor or nurse what kind of tube your loved one has and what each port is for. Write the answers here:

Kind of tube:

Ports:

Used for:

_____

_____

_____

_____

_____

Extra ports can be added to a tube **with adapters.** Ask the doctor or nurse about these.

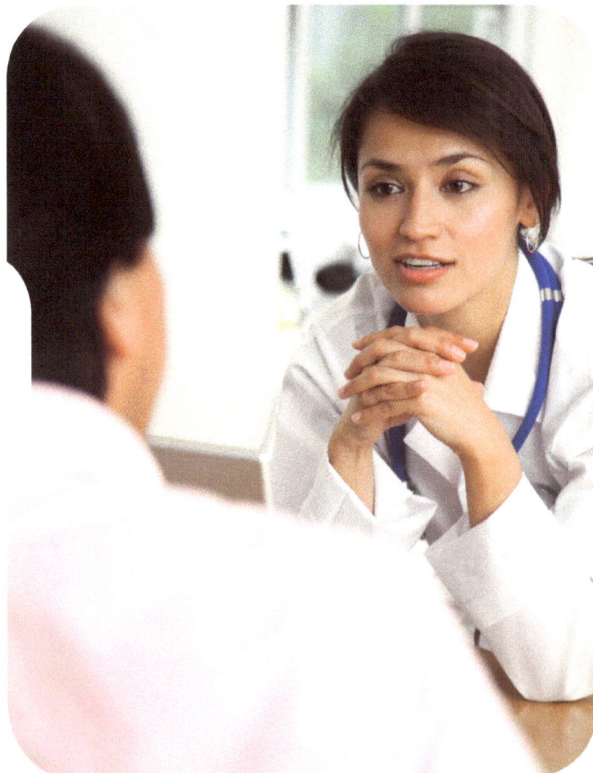

Tube & skin care

Always keep the skin around the stoma clean and dry.

Do these **every day:**

- **Wash hands** with soap and warm water for 30 seconds.

- **Gently wipe the tube and the skin around it.** Use a soft, clean cloth or gauze wet with warm water. If needed, you may use a gentle soap as long as you rinse it off. **(Do not leave gauze under the bumper or around the tube.)** Keep the area uncovered (unless your loved one pulls on the tube) so you will see any leakage.

- **Clean under the bumper** that is against the skin. If needed, use a cotton-tipped swab to clean under the bumper. **Be careful not to pull on the tube.** Gently pat the skin dry with a soft cloth or gauze.

- **Gently turn a G-tube or PEG tube** to keep the balloon or bumper from sticking to one place inside the stomach. **Do not turn or rotate a J-Tube.**

With each feeding, check the skin **for redness, pain or swelling.** Also check for **leakage** or drainage around the tube. If this happens, clean the skin with gauze or a wash cloth, and call the doctor or nurse right away.

If your tube has a balloon, check the amount of water in the balloon weekly.

Gather supplies:

- 4x4 split gauze
- tape
- Qtips®
- saline

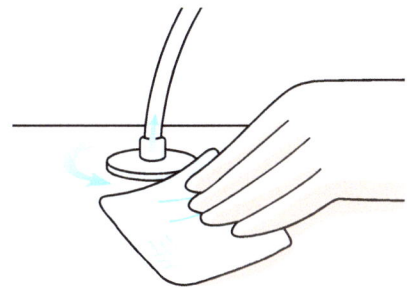

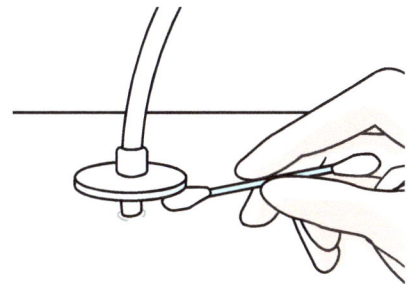

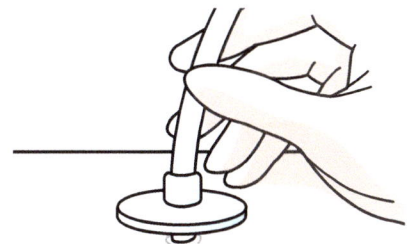

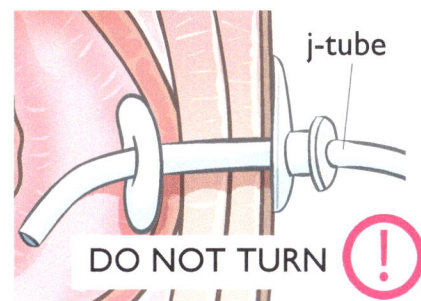

j-tube

DO NOT TURN

Safety checks

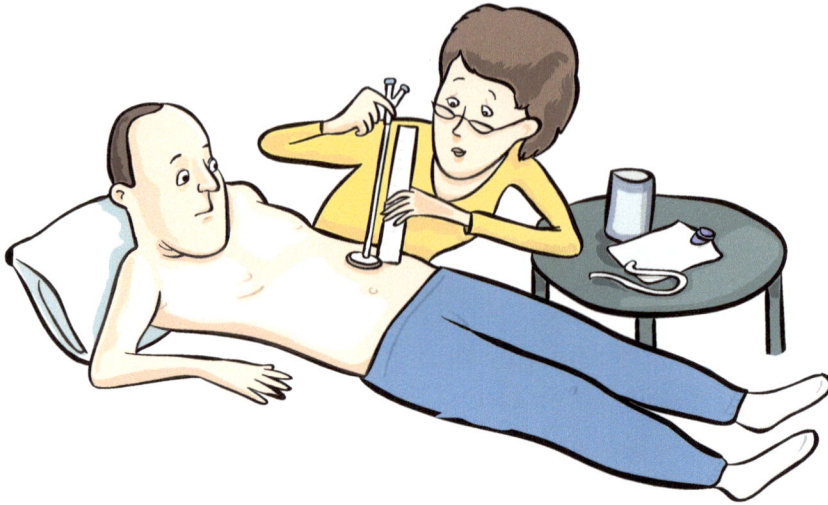

Before starting a feeding—or every 8 hours
if giving a continuous feeding (see page 17)— do these:

1. **Check the tube.** Make sure it is in the right place. Look
   at the length of the tube coming out of the belly. (Either
   measure it, or check the marking on the side of the tube.)
   Making a dark mark on the tubing can be helpful. If the tube
   is shorter or longer than the last time you checked, it moved.
   Stop the feeding and call the doctor or nurse.

2. **Check the bumper.** Make sure it is secure against the
   stomach to keep your tube in place and prevent leakage
   which can irritate the skin. If the bumper is out of place,
   gently pull on the tube until you feel resistance and slide
   the bumper down on the skin.

3. **Check for bleeding.** A few drops of blood from the stoma
   is OK. Call the doctor or nurse if there is:

   • more than a few drops of blood from the stoma

   • blood in the patient's stool

   • coughing up blood

Tell the doctor or nurse what the blood looks like
(bright red, dark brown, etc.)

(Your doctor may choose to skip this step, so be sure to check with him or her.)

4. **Check the stomach.** Be sure the food is moving through and emptying into the small intestine. This is called "checking for residual" (or residue).

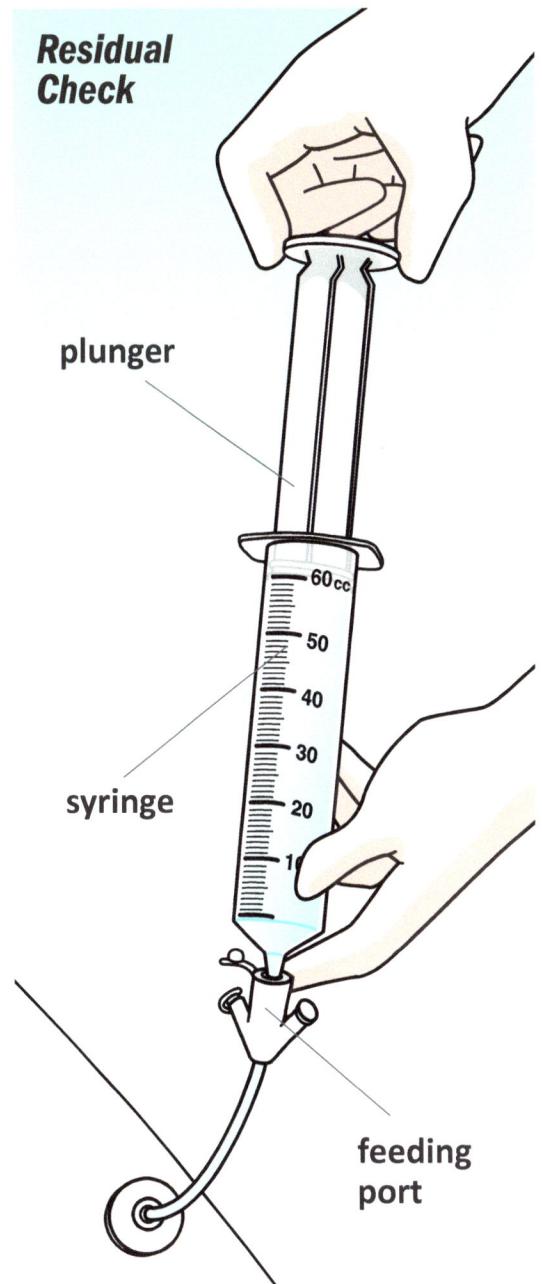

Residual Check

plunger

syringe

60 cc
50
40
30
20
1

feeding port

- If giving continuous feeding, **stop the feeding.**

- Take the feeding bag tube out of the tube feeding port.

- Put a large, catheter-tipped syringe into the feeding port. Gently pull back (withdraw) on the syringe plunger.

- If you are able to withdraw 100 cc or more of the stomach contents, **inject it back into the feeding port.** (You may need 2 syringes or a cup to hold the contents.) Flush the tube with warm water (see page 10). Wait 30 minutes to 1 hour before feeding.

- Then check again to see if the residue is less than 100 cc. If it is, the stomach is emptying the right way. If there is still over 100 cc, call the doctor or nurse.

- **Rinse and flush the syringe with water.**

5. Check the tube for clogging.

Place the end of the syringe in a cup of warm water. Slowly pull back on the plunger.

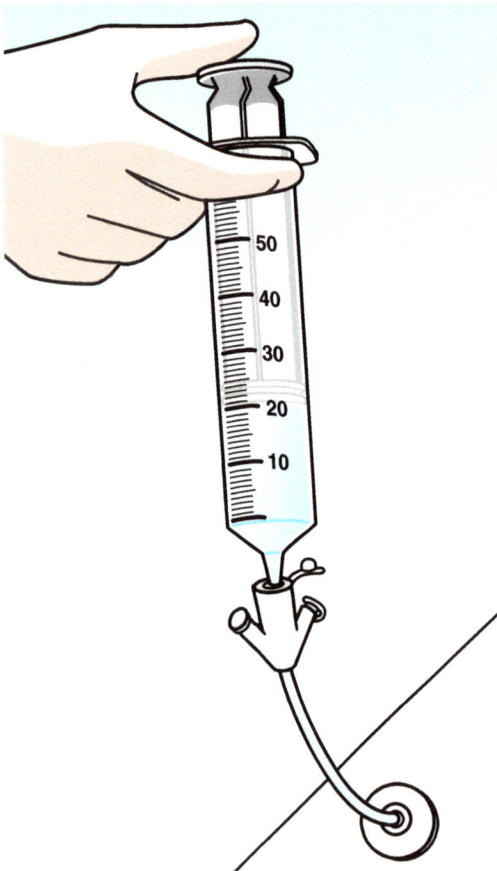

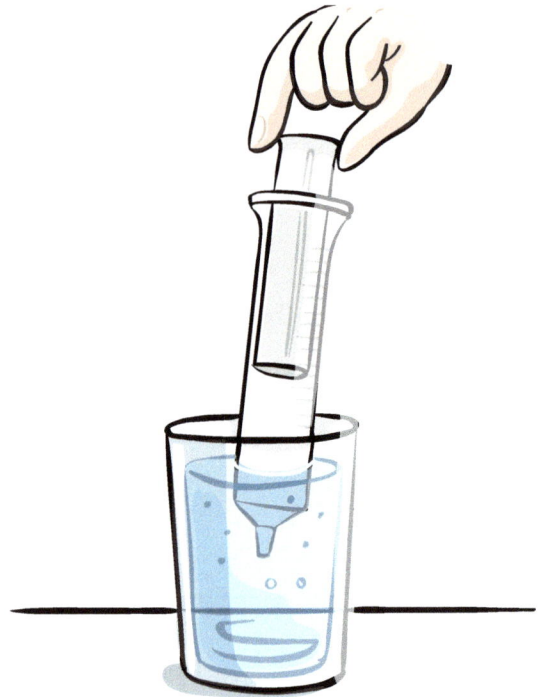

Draw up 15 to 20 cc of warm water into the syringe. Inject it into the feeding port to be sure the tube is clear. (If your doctor has you do residual checks, do that before you check the tube for clogging.)

Flushing

If the tube is clogged, try to clear it.

- Draw up about 15 to 20 cc more of warm water. Inject it into the feeding port.

- If this doesn't work, try to gently massage (rub) the tube to remove any clumps of food. Use one hand to hold the tube firmly at the stoma while you rub the tube.

- If you still can't flush the tube, call the doctor or nurse.

The best way to prevent clogging is to **flush the tube well with warm water before and after every feeding.**

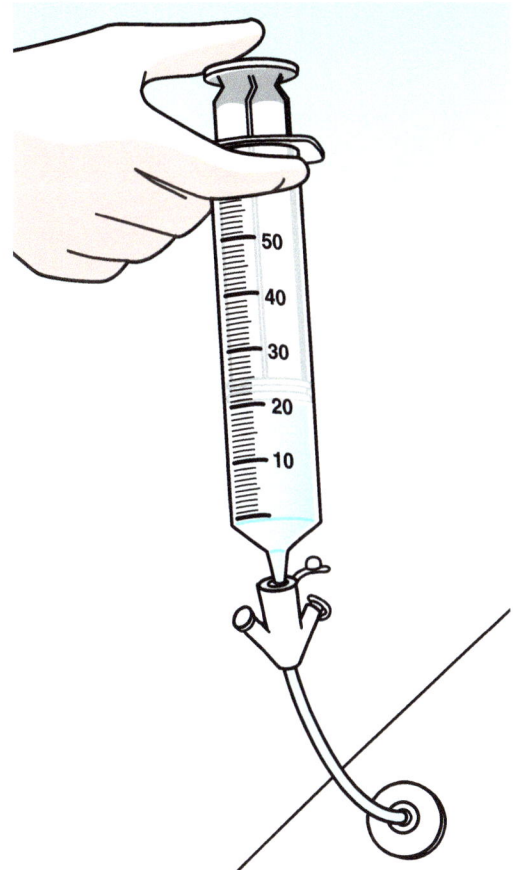

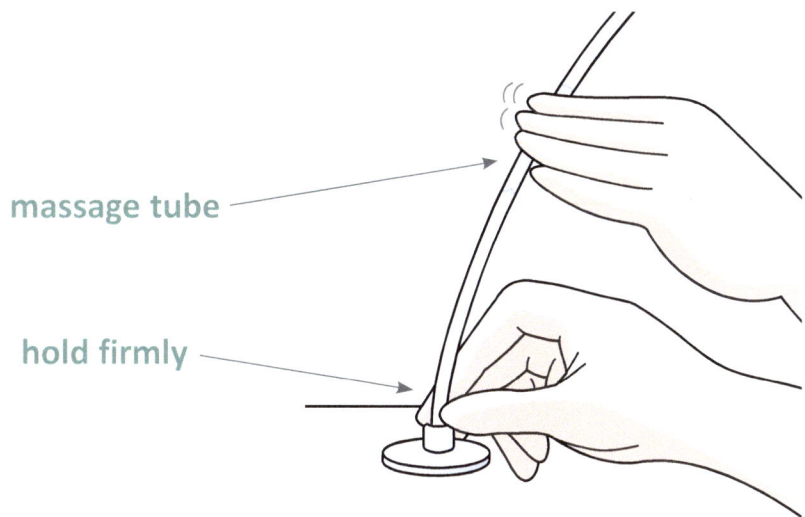

massage tube

hold firmly

Feedings

Make yourself or your loved one as comfortable as you can when feeding. Make sure you are sitting in the right position.

Sit or lie with the head or upper body raised at least 30 degrees (2 to 3 pillows). If you are able to sit up in a chair that would be even better. This will help keep the feeding down and prevent vomiting which can cause you to breathe fluid into your lungs. Never lie down flat during a feeding. With bolus feeding remain with head raised for at least 30 minutes after feeding. If you are receiving a continuous feed, your head should remain elevated at all times.

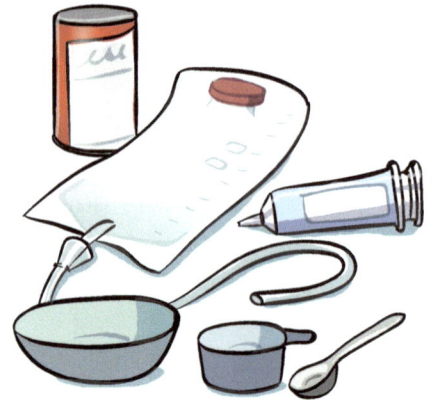

Wash your hands and supplies well. You will need: formula, feeding bag or syringe, bowls, measuring cup, spoons and water.

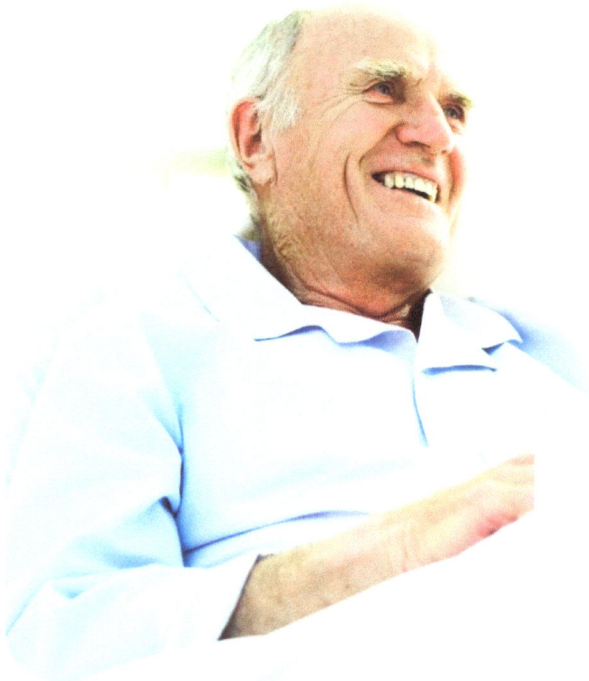

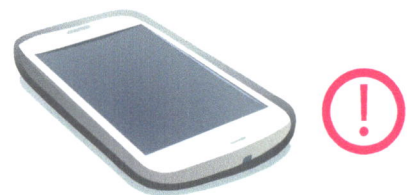

Caution

If your loved one starts to vomit:

1. Turn him on his side right away.
2. Stop the feeding.
3. Prop him up, and lean his head forward.
4. Call the doctor or nurse.

Types of food

The doctor will prescribe the type and amount of food to be given. *The types of food are:

- **premixed (or canned) formula**
  Clean the top of the can with soap and water, and rinse well. Shake it well before opening.

- **powdered formula**
  Follow the directions on the container (or those given by the doctor or dietitian). **Measure the exact amount of water and formula called for.** Mix well with a wire whisk.

- **table food**
  Follow the doctor or dietitian's instructions. Write them here:

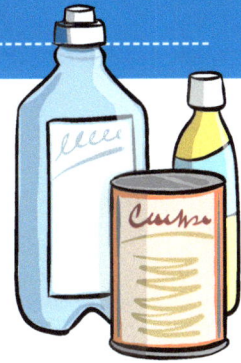

Always store any unused formula in a covered bowl or jar in the refrigerator. **Throw away any formula not used within 24 hours after it is opened or mixed** (even if it has been kept in the refrigerator).

_____

_____

_____

_____

_____

_____

_____

_____

_____

*Check with insurance company to see what types of food are covered.

Types of feedings

Make feeding a social event. Join family or friends at the dinner table if possible. Make feeding as pleasant as you can.

There are **2 ways to feed** through a tube—**bolus and continuous.**

Bolus feeding

This type of feeding is for those who are able to feed themselves or who can handle a large amount of food at one time. It is done 3 or 4 times a day. Most of the time, it takes about **15 to 30 minutes.**

The food is poured into a large syringe or a feeding bag with a tube. A clamp on the tube keeps the food from running through the tube until you are ready.

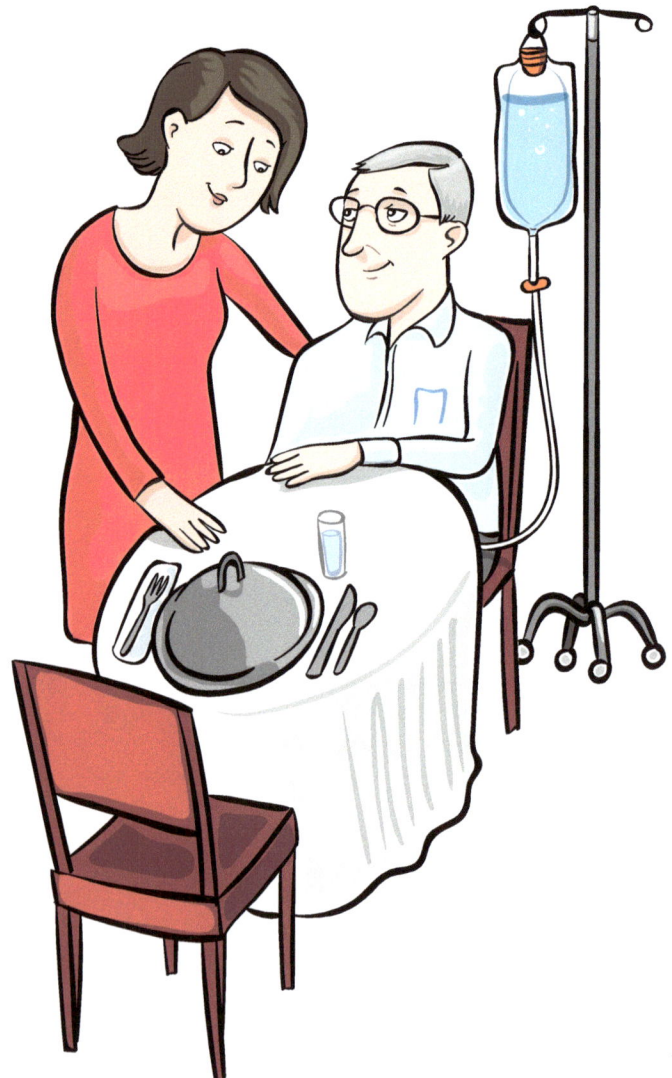

using a syringe

1. Remove the plunger. Put the tip of the syringe
   into the feeding port.

2. Pour the formula into the syringe.

3. Hold the syringe above the stomach. Let the formula
   flow in at a slow rate—over 15 to 30 minutes.

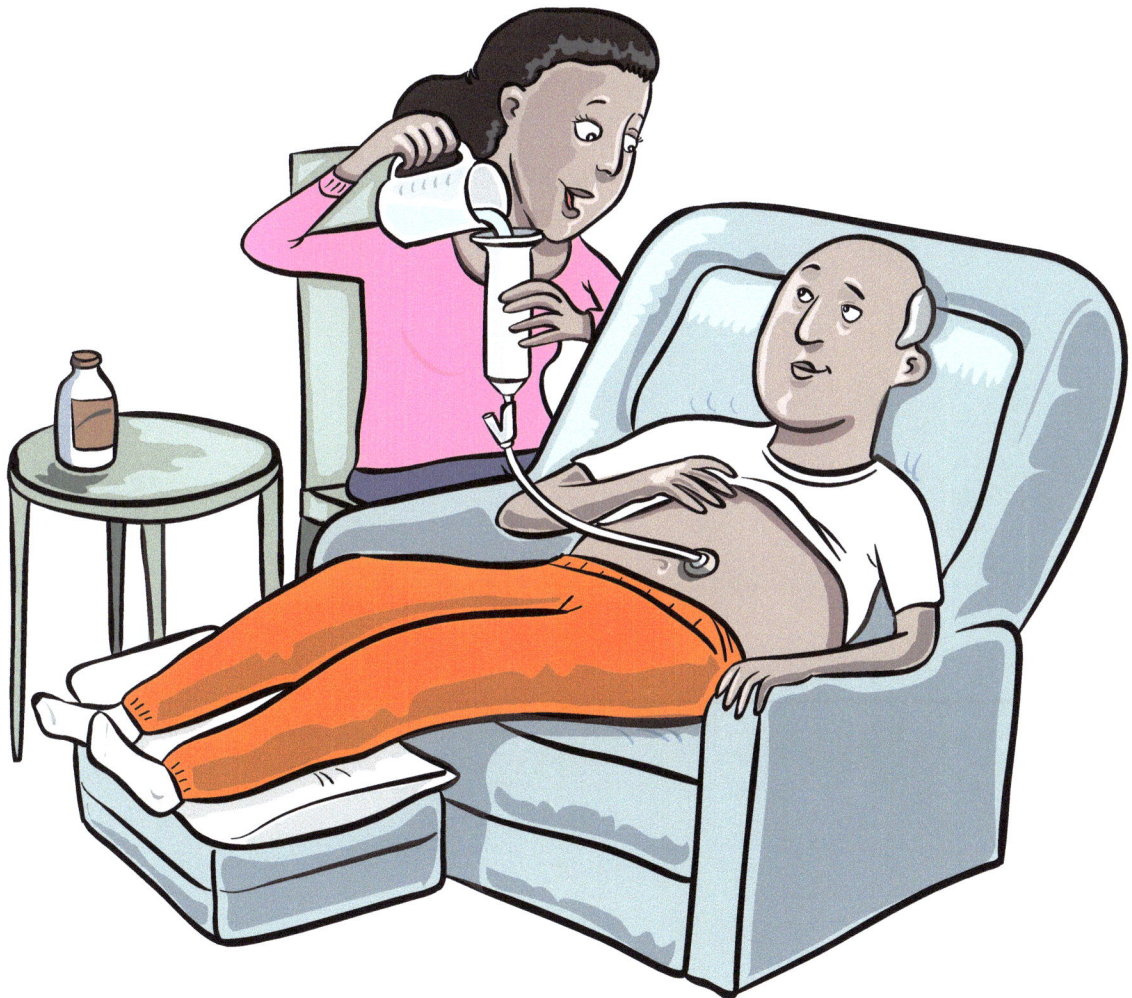

using a feeding bag

1. Pour the formula or food into the feeding bag.

2. Let a small amount run through the feeding bag tube to clear out all the air. (This helps prevent gas.) The food should run through the bag until it begins to come out of the tube.

3. Close the clamp on the feeding bag tube.

4. Place the tip of the feeding bag tube into the feeding tube port. Open the clamp.

5. Hold the feeding bag above the stomach. Let the formula in at a slow rate. You can hang the feeding bag on a wall hook to keep it higher than the stomach. Ask your nurse about other ways to keep the bag above the stomach.

Hold or hang bag about 18 inches higher than the stomach. This will help to reduce cramping.

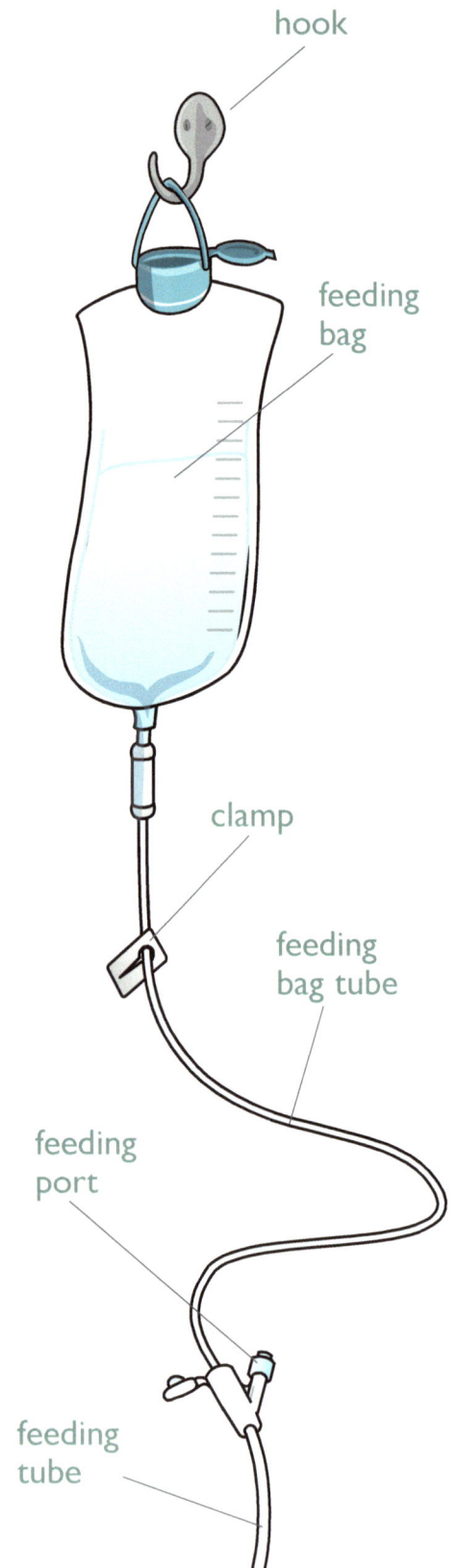

hook

feeding bag

clamp

feeding bag tube

feeding port

feeding tube

After the meal

When the **bolus** feeding is finished:

- Take the feeding bag tube or syringe out of the feeding port.

- **Flush the tube** with warm water (See page 10.)

- Close the cap.

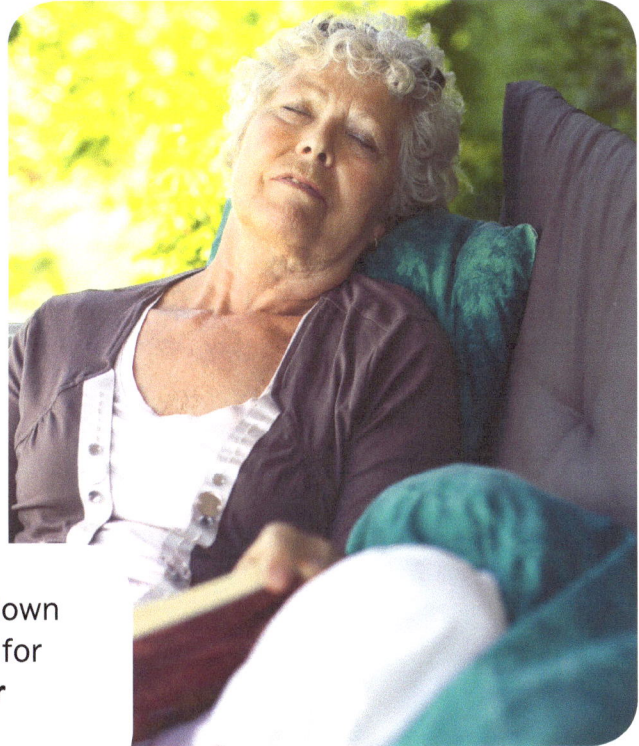

- **Stay seated** or lying down with your head raised for **30 minutes to 1 hour** after the feeding.

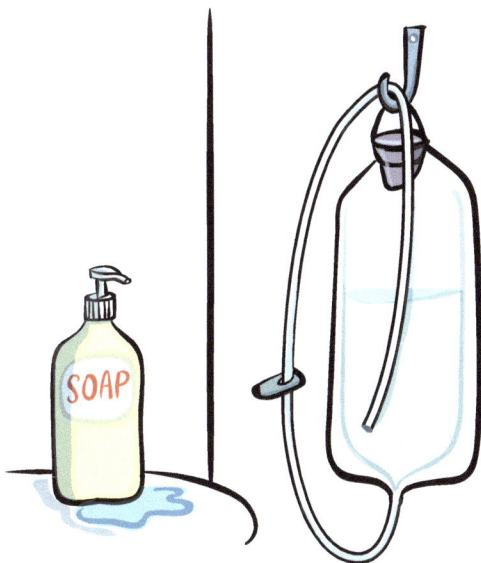

You may be able to reuse the feeding bag and tube. Ask the nurse how often they should be replaced.

If you can reuse the bag and tube:

- Wash them in warm soapy water and rinse well.

- With clamp open, hang to air dry.

- Store in a clean, dry place.

Continuous feeding

This type of feeding is for those who can't take a lot of food at one time. **Food is dripped slowly into the stomach, sometimes all day and night.**

You connect the feeding bag to the feeding port of the tube. The food runs down into the stomach or small intestine. Most of the time a pump is used. This makes the food go in at a slow, steady rate.

1. Turn the pump to stop/off.

2. Close the clamp on the tubing.

3. Pour the formula or food into the feeding bag.

feeding bag

clamp

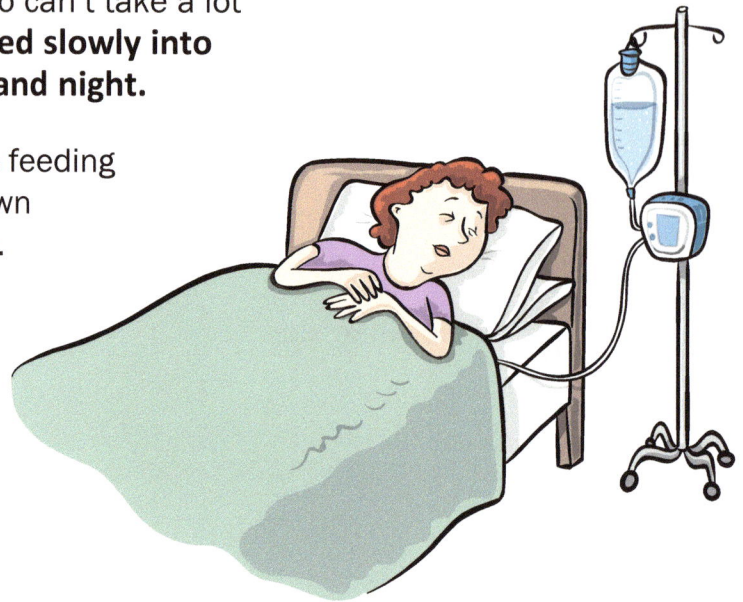

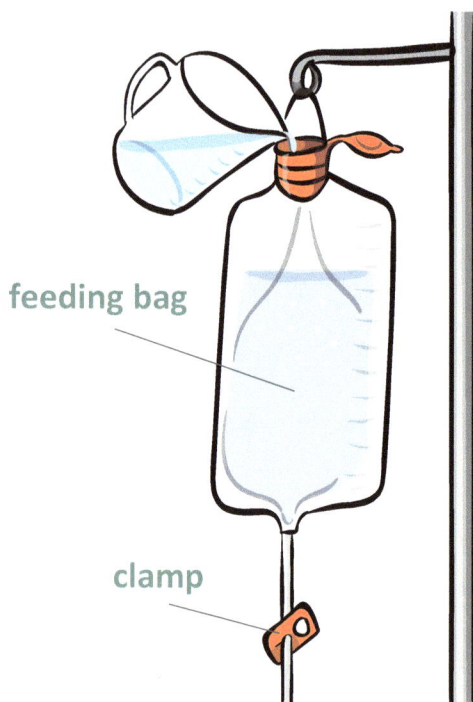

4. Let a small amount run through the feeding bag tube to **clear out all the air.** (This helps prevent gas and problems with the pump.) The food should run through the bag until it begins to come out the tube.

5. **Close the clamp** on the feeding bag tube.

(continued on next page)

6. Set up the pump. (The nurse or someone from the company that supplies the pump will teach you how to do this.)

7. Place the tip of the feeding bag tube into the tube feeding port.

8. **Open the clamp** on the tube.

9. Turn the pump to start/run.

pump

feeding bag tube

feeding port

tube

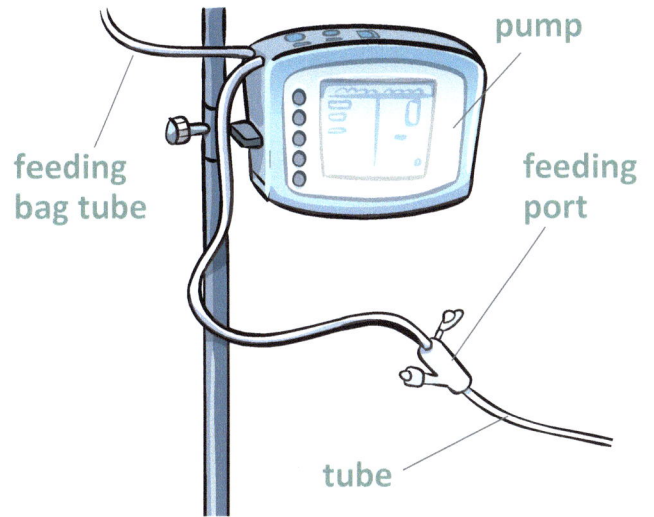

You can make notes on how to set up the pump here:

*Type of pump:*_____

_____

*Rate:*_____

_____

*Start:*_____

_____

*Stop time:*_____

_____

*Amount (cc's)*_____

_____

*Other directions:*_____

_____

_____

_____

_____

flushing with continuous feeding

When giving continuous feeding, flush the feeding tube **every 3 to 4 hours.** This will keep it from getting clogged.

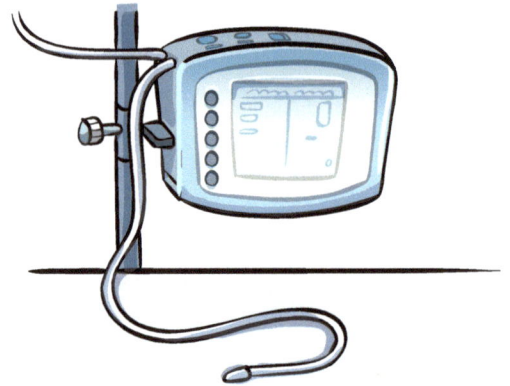

1. **Stop the feeding.** (Turn the pump off or to "hold".)

2. Draw up 50 to 75 cc (or the amount your doctor tells you) of **warm water** into the syringe.

3. Take the feeding bag tube out of the tube feeding port. Pinch the tubing so the food won't flow out. (Hold ports higher than stomach.)

4. Inject the water into the feeding port. Make sure the tube is clear.

5. If the tube is clear, connect the feeding bag tube back to the feeding port of the tube.

6. Turn the pump back on. (Or turn from "hold" back to "run".)

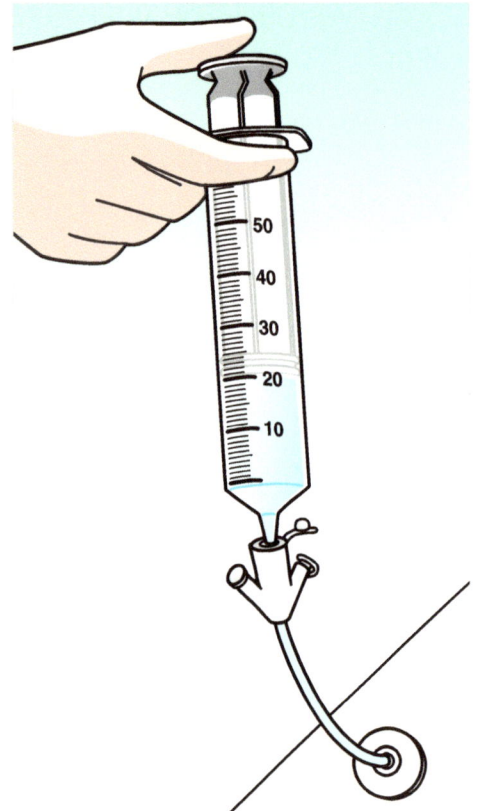

Ask the nurse how often the bag and tube should be replaced.

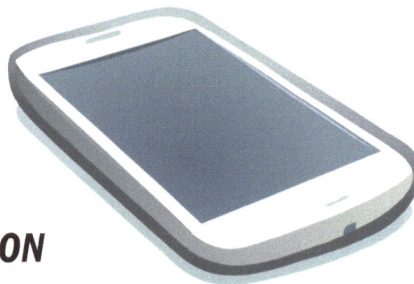

⚠ CAUTION

If you can't flush the tube, do not reconnect the tubes. Call the doctor or nurse.

Medicines

Ask for medicines in liquid or patch form. If a medicine only comes in pill form, **ask the pharmacist if it's OK to crush them.** If so, crush and dissolve them in 50 cc (about 3 tablespoons) of warm water—one medicine at a time. **Never crush enteric coated* or time-released capsules.**

Before you give over-the-counter medicines, ask the doctor or nurse if they are OK for someone with a tube.

Give medicines at the times the doctor tells you to. Ask the doctor if some or all medicines can be dissolved and given at the same time.

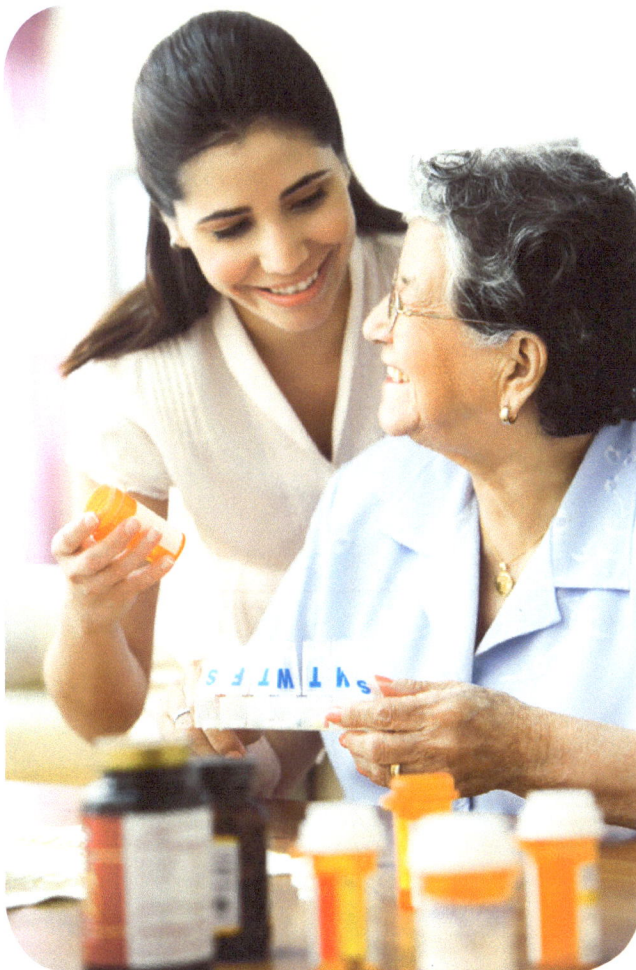

CAUTION (!)

If more than one medicine is to be given at the same time, flush the tube with 10 to 15 cc of warm water **between** medicines. After giving **all** medicines, flush the tube with 30 cc of warm water. If medicine is mixed with formula, it can cause diarrhea. **Stop feeding one hour before and after Dilantin®** (Phenytonin).

*medicine that is coated does not dissolve in the stomach

1. **Make sure all liquids are at room temperature.** Pouring cold liquid into the stomach can cause cramping.

2. Make sure you are in a **sitting position of 30 degrees** (2 to 3 pillows). If you are active and able to stand that is fine too.

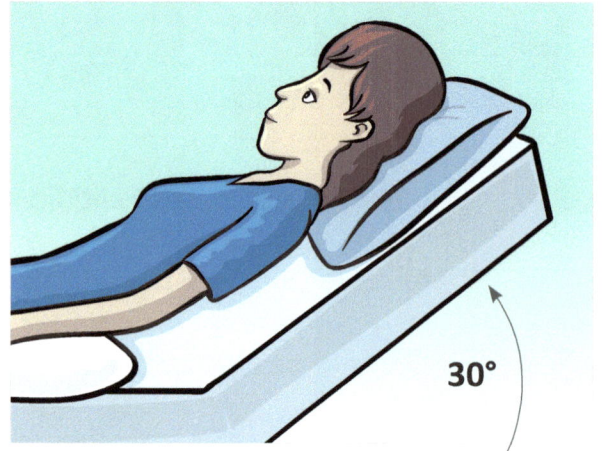

3. Use the medicine port if your feeding tube has one. If using the feeding port for medicines, first flush it with 30 cc of warm water (See page 10.)

4. Pour medicine into a cup so that you can draw it into the syringe.

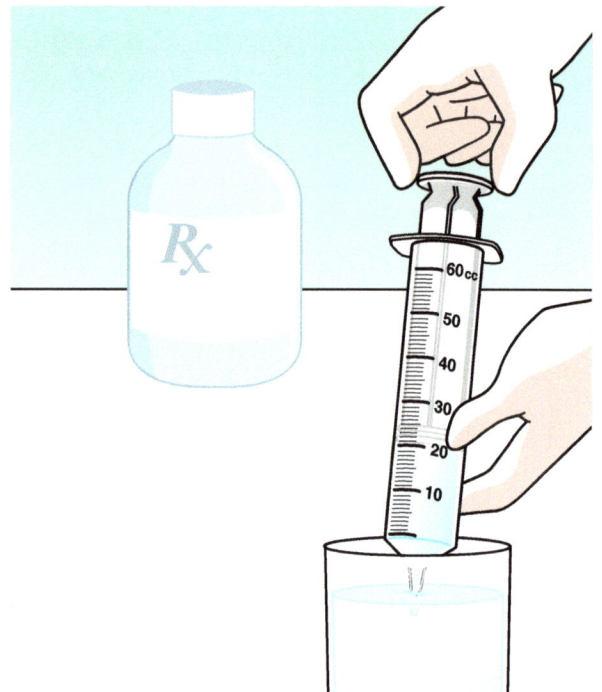

5. Draw up the medicine, and inject it into the feeding or medicine port.

6. Remove the syringe.

7. **Flush the tube** with 30 cc of warm water.

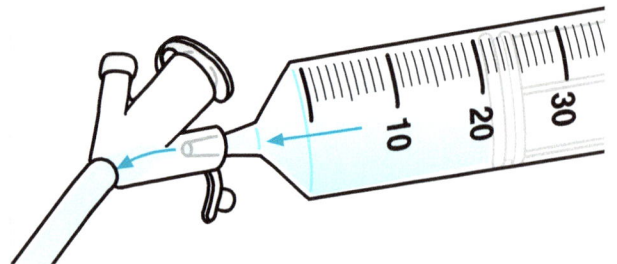

Side effects

Sore mouth

Even if you are not eating, your mouth needs care to keep it from getting sore. Brush and rinse every day. Using a lip balm or product such as Chapstick® or Vaseline® to help keep lips moist.

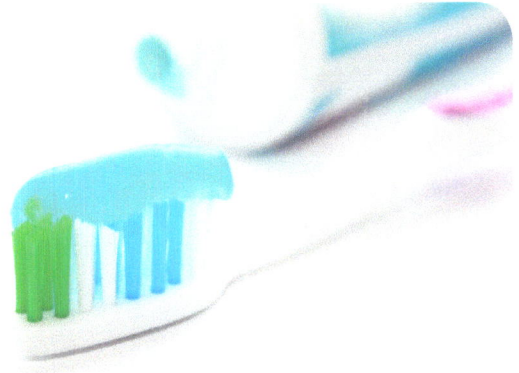

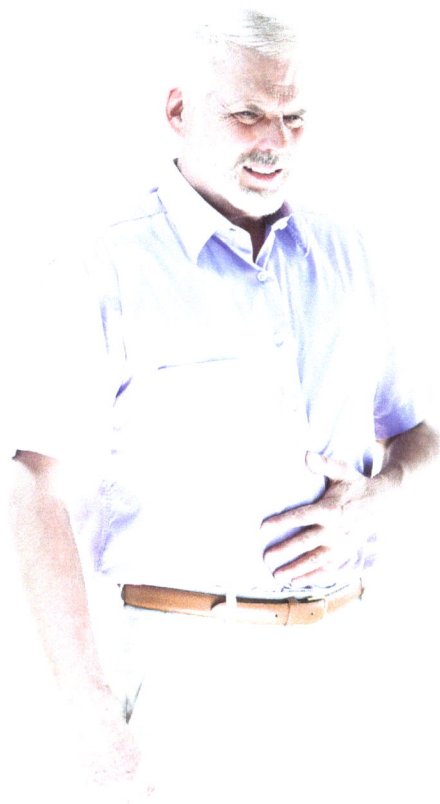

Gas or upset stomach

Bolus feeding

If you have a lot of gas or nausea, do not force a feeding. Wait until you no longer feel full or sick. If you miss more than one feeding because of this, call the doctor or nurse.

Continuous feeding

If you are feeling full or sick, stop the feeding, and flush the tube. Or slow the feeding down (by setting the pump at a slower rate) for 1 to 2 hours. When you no longer feel full or sick, start the feeding again. Call the doctor or nurse if this problem lasts for more than 4 to 6 hours.

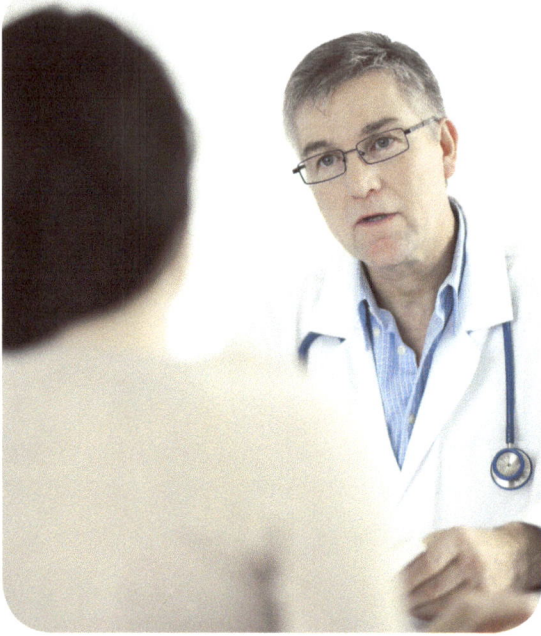

Diarrhea

Diarrhea is frequent, loose, watery stools. If this lasts for more than two days, call the doctor or nurse. Sometimes diarrhea is caused by:

- the rate the formula goes in.

- the type of formula. Ask your nurse if you need to change types.

- formula that has gone bad. Throw away the formula, feeding bag and tube after 24 hours (unless your doctor or nurse says you can reuse them).

Constipation

Constipation is having fewer stools than normal or stools that are very hard and may hurt to pass. Sometimes you need to give more water, or give prune juice through the tube to soften the stool. **If constipation lasts for more than 5 days or there is no stool for 3 days, call the doctor or nurse.**

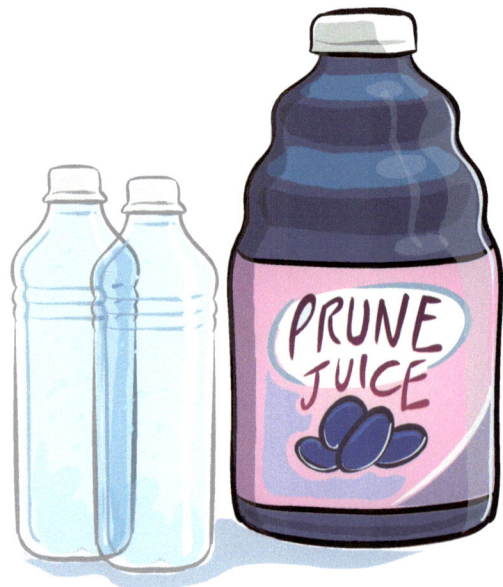

When to call the doctor

Call your doctor immediately:

- if you see redness, drainage or swelling around the tube site.

- if you are bleeding through the tube, coughing up blood or see blood in your stool.

- if the tube comes out or becomes clogged, and you can't clear it by flushing.

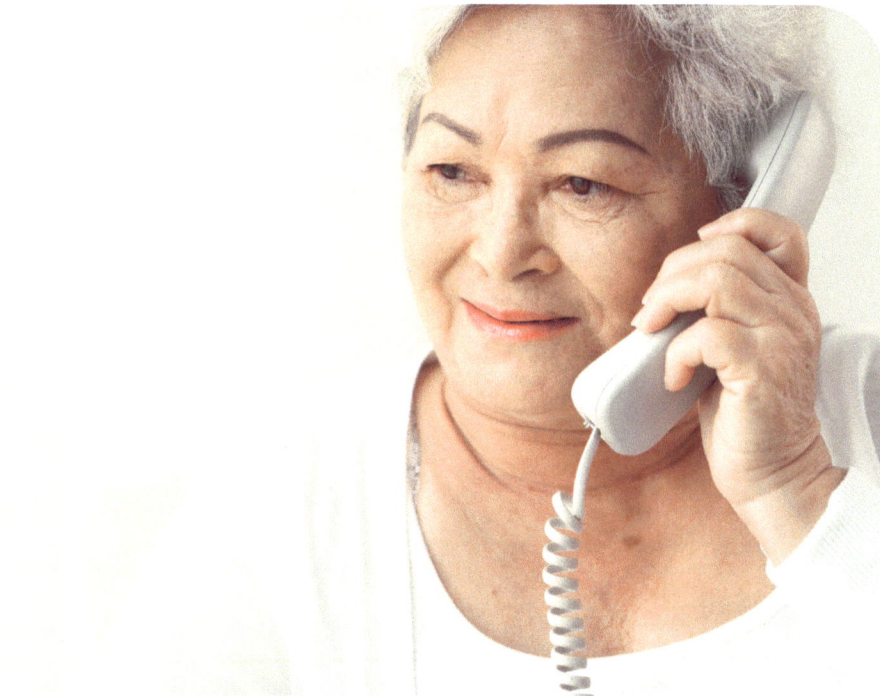

*Doctor:*_____ *Phone #:*_____

*Nurse:*_____ *Phone #:*_____

Notes

---

www.ingramcontent.com/pod-product-compliance
Lightning Source LLC
Chambersburg PA
CBHW060857270326
41934CB00003B/182